*What You Think and Say,
How You Dine and What You Eat
Shows Who You Are*

What You Think and Say

How You Dine and What You Eat

Shows Who You Are

*The Word of God for us,
revealed through the
cherub of divine Wisdom,
Brother Emanuel*

*Given through the prophetess
of the Lord,
Gabriele– Würzburg*

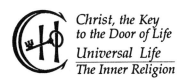

Christ, the Key
to the Door of Life
Universal Life
The Inner Religion

Gabriele Publishing House
P.O. Box 2221, Deering, NH 03244
(844) 576-0937
WhatsApp/Messenger: +49 151 1883 8742
www.Gabriele-Publishing-House.com

First Edition, 1997

Published by:
© Universal Life
The Inner Religion
PO Box 3549
Woodbridge, CT 06525
U S A

Licensed edition
translated from the original German title:
"Was Du denkst und sprichst, wie Du speist
und was Du ist zeigt wer Du bist".

Order No. S135en

From the Universal Life Series
with the consent of
© Verlag DAS WORT GmbH
im Universellen Leben
Max-Braun-Strasse 2
97828 Marktheidenfeld/Altfeld
Germany

The German edition is the work of reference for all
questions regarding the meaning of the contents

ISBN 3-890841-02-1

The Word of God for us,
revealed through the
cherub of divine Wisdom,
Brother Emanuel.

Given through the prophetess
of the Lord,
Gabriele – Würzburg

Preface

The two small books *"What You Think and Say Shows Who You Are"* and *"How You Dine and What You Eat Shows Who You Are"* are now combined into one book.

These plain volumes, given to us by way of the divine Wisdom, contain spiritual instructions seldom found in such a simple and condensed form which is at the same time appealing, loving and stimulating. On each page, we can read about how to sense and fathom life in all its fullness, beginning with its external, everyday appearance. We receive impulses and help towards a higher quality of life. In this way, we may come to know and understand ourselves better — as well as our neighbor. On the path of self-recognition and purification, we draw ever closer to our eternal being, which is beauty, clarity, righteousness, kindness, selflessness and peace.

You will find numerous repetitions in this book. They are not slipped into it by chance. The person who reads this text attentively will realize that in his explanations the spirit teacher and cherub of divine Wisdom, Brother Emanuel, is repeatedly shedding light from different perspectives on human events, on spiritual laws and principles, as well as on possibilities for self-recognition on the path to spirituality. In this way, the teaching and helping Spirit of God touches different aspects and vibration fields of the human consciousness, so that what He wants to explain to us can take root in us. Our human way of learning is thus taken into consideration by repeatedly addressing our consciousness with different spiritual impulses all pointing in the same direction.

From the spiritual point of view, collecting knowledge is of little use to us. It is only the application, the practical application in our everyday life — that is, the actualization of what we have recognized — that brings us spiritual gain. Then we leave the superficiality of an externalized life. We begin to fulfill the divine laws more and more, to comprehend the life, the truth, the divine in all things and to move within them.

Würzburg, July 1997

The Original Christians
in Universelles Leben

What You Think
and Say
Shows Who You Are

The Consciousness, God,
is eternally being

God is love.

God is eternal symphony.

God is harmony.

God is peace.

The consciousness, God, is eternally being.

All pure forms of Being are contained in the consciousness, God. The essence of the kingdoms of nature and of the stars, the pure beings and the pure in soul and man constitute the consciousness, God.

Everything that is came forth from love, God, since God is love. Everything which will be, will come forth from love, God, because God is eternal love and wisdom.

Nothing which is can exist without God, the love, which is the life.

Nothing is outside of God. God is All in all things. God is omnipresent Spirit, all-effective.

God is the universal, absolute law.

God is all-ruling.

The law, God, is irrefutable. The one who lives the law, lives God, and God lives through him.

God is love

The one who lives God, the law, lives the high power of absolute love. He has thereby become the law himself, which is God, the love.

God, the love and the life, the peace and the harmony, lives more and more each day through the soul, through the person, who is on the path to the Absolute, to God, the law of life.

The one who includes God, the selfless love, in his feeling, thinking, speaking and acting becomes wise. In the course of his spiritual life, he will become the law itself. He feels, thinks and speaks from the law of love, for he has become selfless love, impersonal, spirit of His spirit. He is divine again, just as God, the love, has created him. All souls have to walk this path one day, because the spiritual body is immortal. It came forth from the source of life, out of the love, God, and will return to the source, the wellspring, the love, because the pure being is divine and at the same time the law.

The pure spirit body is compressed law, God. When the soul of a person finds its way back to its origin, to the love, to God, it has become again the immaculate spiritual body. The spirit body in the person is then consciously divine again, the law itself. The spirit in the spirit body and in the person feels, thinks and speaks divinely, absolutely. This means, the incarnate spirit being, the spirit being in the person, is again divine. Spirit being and person are divine.

The one who allows God to become effective in him, by actualizing the eternal laws, lives in fulfillment more and more. He becomes meek and humble of heart. His nature and appearance will come to resemble the love of God. His world of feelings and thoughts becomes selfless love. The words of the person will then also be kind, just as his nature has become.

The thoughts and actions of such a person rest on the foundation of divine love, for his world of feelings and thoughts is love, selflessness. The words and the behavior of this person then build upon his world of selfless feelings and thoughts.

When the foundation, the world of feelings and thoughts of a person, is not selfless love, then his words and deeds will be effective for only a short time — for as long as they bear and maintain the outer world of appearance, into which feelings, thoughts, words and deeds were projected.

And so, what man thinks and says, is what he is

If a person's world of feelings and thoughts is far from God, the love, harmony and peace, then he is focused primarily on himself. He is oriented to his body and not to the whole; he is not aligned with the consciousness, God. His human will, which is active as projection and production in the external world, is conditioned by time alone and is therefore relative. It is not capable of living for long, because matter is only short-lived.

And so, when a person's world of feelings and thoughts is small, focused only on himself and his immediate surroundings, then his all-consciousness is narrow and dis-

13

turbed. It is superimposed with human wants and longings.

People who think only of themselves and their immediate surroundings are self-centered. Often they are hardhearted when their desires and ways of thinking are not fulfilled.

The reasons for hard-heartedness and intolerance are human sensations and thoughts, man's ego, which has placed itself into the very center of material life.

People whose spirit-awareness is extremely narrow and overlaid live predominantly in body-awareness. That is, they are oriented to physical things.

People who are oriented only to their bodies want to compensate for the divine wisdom they have lost by means of intellectual living, with their way of feeling, thinking, speaking and acting. Since they are impoverished in their inner being by the shadowing of their souls, all their aspiration is to display to the world what they no longer possess, namely, divine wisdom.

The one who is oriented to the world is the one who is oriented to his body, who thinks only of his interests and acts accordingly. His nature is usually hard-hearted. He is frustrated and coarser in his structure than people who strive towards inner wisdom. He reacts extremely sensitively when his ideas and his field of knowledge, which are his whole pride, are questioned.

And so, if a person's way of thinking, speaking and acting focuses only on his own person and perhaps on the small circle around him, on the few people who have a similar

14

way of thinking, who are a part of his field of vision, he will fight with thoughts, words and deeds everything that is not his own, which does not correspond to his egoism. In his feelings and thoughts, he is then against everyone and everything which is of no use to his ego and is not necessary for his egotistical way of thinking and living. People with a strong ego also have a harsh facial expression.

Every person betrays his feeling, thinking and acting through his facial expressions and gestures, by the way he moves his body.

What a person feels and thinks has an effect on his entire posture.

The spiritual body, the soul, has magnetic fields.

The soul, which is the book of life, registers the positive feelings, thoughts and deeds of the person, as well as his unlawful life, his egotistical behavior. The one as well as the other is reflected on the person. The body is the expression of what a person feels, thinks and speaks, of what he actually is.

The egotistical person is moody. His mood can even develop into brutality. He wants to be right in everything he thinks and says. He fights for "his" right, because justice has become shadowed through his egotistical life. Therefore, his intellect is the measure of all things and the master of his ego.

The selfless person who lives from the law, whose basis is selfless love, is meek and humble. He is not a know-it-all. He will give, explain and love, by turning the other cheek when his neighbor wants to keep his own opinion. This means he will not argue with him, but will let justice prevail, by knowing the measure of all things and communicating as much of it as his neighbor is capable of understanding. He will leave him his free will in thoughts and actions, as long as his way of thinking and acting does not harm his fellow man. He will not be silent when injustice is done. He will speak and act from the law, but will neither overload his neighbor nor overwhelm him with his answers.

The human body is, like every form, an energy-body, an energy potential which radiates and vibrates in accordance with the feelings, thoughts and deeds of the individual.

Each person radiates what he is, what he has felt, thought and spoken towards himself. A person's conduct also molds his inner and outer nature.

The one who does not strive for the absolute, the pure, the selfless, the divine love, peace and harmony, the powers which dwell within every soul, will emit only disharmony.

People who live in the awareness of their body, who live selfishly and not in the awareness of the whole, live in their own small world. Their consciousness is narrow and overlaid by their way of thinking and acting.

Each person emits what he is; for soul and person are simultaneously sender and receiver. Imperceptibly, a person emits who he is and imperceptibly he attracts, in turn, the same. He receives back what he emits or sends out, for like always attracts like.

Everyone who approaches the zone of vibration, the thought-complexes, of the human ego, will be influenced by them more or less, according to how the soul of the one who approaches his neighbor is burdened.

When the soul of a person is similarly burdened as the person who influences him, soul and person will take in what his neighbor sends out in the form of opinions, ideas and desires.

One receives from the other, because he thinks and feels similarly, because his energy-body vibrates like his neighbor's. Thus, he makes the opinions and ideas of his neighbor his own; he becomes an imitator.

People with strong egotistical inclinations, who are oriented only to material things, mold and shape their environment according to their will. They impose their will upon everyone who lives in their surroundings and submits to their will.

Only those people will submit to their neighbor's self-will who, in their world of sensations and thoughts, vibrate similarly to the one who wants to shape his environment according to his will.

In accordance with his origin, every human being is divine, for God is love, peace and harmony. The nature of our heavenly Father is absolute, selfless and always giving. God, the law, is not the ego of the person, but the I Am of the soul, the absolute, the incorruptible core of the being, which is continuously active and indestructible.

The incorruptible core of the being, God, the love, in soul and person, gives unceasingly.

The eternal law, God, is far from the terms of "mine" and "me," or "I am my own best friend."

God created His child, the pure being of the heavens, in His image. His child, the divine being, bears within itself the divine aspects of love, peace and harmony, the selfless, eternally giving aspects, God. In the innermost being of every person is the pure spirit body, the child of God. As long as this spirit being in the person is burdened, it is called a soul.

As long as a person is oriented to this world, he cannot live a God-conscious life. The result is that he cannot recognize his heritage, the All-consciousness, the essence of all life, and therefore cannot let it become active.

The All-consciousness, God, the love and wisdom, is at the same time creation-consciousness, since the love gives continuously. The one who draws near to the All-consciousness, God, will give selflessly and develop in himself all the aspects of his heritage: love, wisdom, kindness, peace and harmony.

If the creation forces of God — love, wisdom, kindness, peace and harmony — are covered over, if they are layered over by wrong egotistical feeling, thinking, speaking and acting, then the person becomes cumbersome in his way of thinking, more and more oriented to the earth, and the soul, more and more tied to the earth.

People who think only of themselves and who criticize their neighbor constantly, who accept and receive only their own self and reject their neighbor because he might oppose their convictions, have to ask themselves sooner or later who or what they are.

Everything is radiation

And so, a person radiates his own way of feeling, thinking and acting. Therefore, you are your sensations; you, yourself, are your words and actions. Your body and your soul radiate what you are.

You are a body of thought. You are your own world of thoughts. It is in you, on you and around you. You radiate who you are.

You constantly portray your own nature — clearly visible to the neighbor who lives near the All-consciousness. Egotistical sensations and thoughts are never divine sensations and thoughts. Hard-hearted, brutal words never flow from the divine selfless love, the inner harmony and divine peace. Man, himself, has inflicted hard-heartedness on himself, by means of feeling, thinking and speaking in the wrong way.

Every deviation from the selfless eternal law of love is egotism. The human ego focuses only on human desires and human matters. The one who thinks only of himself is spun into his world of thoughts, into his base ego.

This egotistical thinking and living shapes the person; it is his body structure. A rough, coarse structure can, in turn, radiate only rude words, hard-hearted sensations, exactly that which lies and is active in the person, in the soul, what the person felt, thought and spoke into himself.

What you are marks you

A fine body structure shows noble features; the person has a noble, selfless conduct. His body rhythm is harmonious and balanced. This becomes evident in his harmonious gestures. His whole being radiates an inner symphony of divine peace and deep stillness. Whatever this person accomplishes is carried out with ease and liveliness, for he is far from his base ego. He knows and lives his true self. Whatever he touches and holds in his hand, his actions are borne by inner harmony. His whole being is well-balanced.

The behavior of such a person bears witness of his high convictions; his body is well-balanced; his features are beautiful. His world of sensations and thoughts is pure because his inner being has become pure. His words are selfless, not hurtful, but borne by selfless love.

Everything such a noble person accomplishes is carried out from within, because his being is noble and kind. His life is in order and his cast of mind is irreproachable. He is morally faultless. And so, the world of sensations and thoughts of the person is his radiation; it is his structure.

The one who recognizes himself also recognizes his neighbor. The one who lives only in his world of earthly sensations and thoughts is self-centered and not all-conscious, oriented to God. He will never know his neighbor, because he does not know himself. People who think about themselves a lot, whose world of thoughts is trapped in thoughts of possession and desires, who think only about how to increase their possessions and how to fulfill their wishes, are self-centered and become hard-hearted. The hard-heartedness of the personal ego shows itself in its words, in its way of talking, in its gestures, in its affected behavior and conduct.

O man, if you want to know yourself, then observe yourself, what you feel, what you think, how you speak. When your words are rough, when you use ugly words and strong language, then you can recognize your nature in this.

And so, you recognize yourself. Your structure is coarse. As your structure is, so is the make-up of your soul: layered over by egotistical thinking and vain delusion.

If someone is a controlling person, he should examine his words, how he expresses his decisiveness, whether tolerance or intolerance resounds in his words.

0 man, recognize yourself in how you approach your neighbor: Do you accept your neighbor? Are you tolerant or do you reject him? Do you cut off any chance for communication?

Examine yourself, for in this way you can recognize yourself and know who you are.

Are you at odds with your fellow man, your neighbor, with your fellow workers? Examine yourself, what is the nature of the disagreement?

Your neighbor, your fellow worker, is not what you take him to be, but you, yourself, are as you see him, insofar as you criticize him again and again and are irritated by his words and behavior. You see in him only what you either still bear in yourself or what you do not have, but would like to acquire for yourself.

What you think about your neighbor, how you talk about him, tells who you are. Your neighbor is your own mirror.

If you dislike the characteristics and conduct of your neighbor, his words and behavior, his facial expressions, his disharmonious and provoking manner of speaking, and if this irritates you, then examine yourself.

Why does your neighbor irritate you? Recognize yourself in your annoyance; for the same or like thing is in you.

A guilty conscience towards your neighbor, possessiveness or envy may also trigger your irritation. What you think at the moment you meet your neighbor is not necessarily the cause.

That thought may only be an offshoot of the cause, which lies deeper in you. Explore yourself, entrust yourself to the eternal law and become free from yourself, from your base ego.

And so, when you are indignant about your neighbor or even annoyed with him, then he has touched a sore spot in you with his gestures, his facial expressions, his way of talking and the like.

He has stirred up a correspondence within you, causing an energy field to vibrate which triggered similar sensations and thoughts, that is, resonances, in you.

For example, if you are irritated by your neighbor's facial expressions, you can be sure that he has caused a correspondence in you to vibrate. Examine whether you sense that he saw through you, that perhaps he recognized and uncovered what you wanted to hide and not admit to.

Or it may be that you envy his nature or his character traits, because there is something about him which you do not have, but would like to have. In this case, do not examine merely your thoughts and words, but go deeper. Your world of sensations tells you more than your thoughts and words.

A person can recognize himself in many different ways. Every irritation about your neighbor, and every unpleasantness, shows that the same or the like is in you, or that you envy the other for what you do not have. For example, if a person's way of speaking, the harshness of his words, or maybe the disharmonious radiation of his nature irritate you, you have to ask yourself: What was it that reacted in me? Undoubtedly the same or similar qualities.

For instance, if you expect more love from your neighbor, ask yourself why. If you would have enough radiating selfless love yourself, you would let it stream forth, without asking and wondering why your neighbor does not have enough love. And so, when you talk about the lack of love in your neighbor, you have to admit to yourself that you have too little love.

If your intentions are to possess and to have, then you only want to take and not give. Here again you can take measure of your inner being. If you are possessive, you are impoverished within, that is, you have little wisdom or divine energy. Examine yourself and be honest with yourself, and then you will recognize who you are.

The person who has a constant attitude of expectation is oriented towards taking. When through this he reaps the same or the like that corresponds to his own nature, that is, harshness, disharmony, malicious gossip and the like, he can again recognize himself in his irritation.

Every human being is transmitter and receiver at the same time. The one who has an attitude of expectation is attuned to receiving. He is then hit only by what is in him as correspondences and related qualities. He gets upset over people who have what he does not have, or who touch his ego, that is, those thought patterns which he does not want to admit to and which show him his true nature, the way he is.

Both have to be taken into consideration, the related qualities which say that *similar* qualities are present, or the correspondence which says that the *same* qualities and individual character traits are present.

The one who lives in this inner turmoil, whose consciousness and subconscious are dispolarized by egotistical thinking and acting, does not live himself. He is a split personality who lives under diverse influences, and is thus a puppet of those people who irritate him, whom he wants to imitate. And at the same time, he is a puppet of various energy fields outside the earth's atmosphere.

The one who lives in this state of discord ultimately has to say to himself: I am irritated by my own correspondences. So the one who is annoyed by others bears the same or similar traits in himself: harshness and unkindness.

What a person expects of his neighbor is what he himself does not have. Whatever irritates him, the same or the like is in him.

The Almighty Power, God, gives

God, the life, the love, does not have an attitude of expectation, since the Almighty possesses everything that vibrates and lives in infinity.

An attitude of expectation is possessive. The person who lives in this attitude of expectation expects something from his neighbor. In reality, he should expect it of himself! When he has attained it, then he can give.

If you expect love, possessions and goods from your neighbor, then develop love within yourself first, so that you can give selfless love. When you give selfless love, everything you need — and beyond that — will flow towards you. Then you will no longer have to expect it, you already have it.

The one who gives selfless love, who serves selflessly, will receive inner strength, as well as material things, the very things he needs as a human being, and beyond that.

Recognize: All the treasures of infinity are within you.

When you become selfless, oriented solely towards the good, the divine, then the forces, the treasures, of infinity will be manifest in you. The inner fullness, your spiritual consciousness, will begin to vibrate more intensively and will, externally, put everything in order and supply what you need, and beyond that.

Only the one who is poor in his inner being is externally poor. But if you are rich in your inner being, filled with the life, with God, then you will also have what you need in your outer life, and beyond that. For this reason, O man, look first at the beam in your own eye and remove it, so that you can truly recognize the splinter in your neighbor's eye in the right way, and be able to serve and help him so that he, too, may recognize and remove it.

A person can be a good, selfless teacher and servant to his neighbor only when he has conquered himself and speaks not only on the basis of his correspondences, but draws and gives from the treasure of rich experience, from what he has lived and gone through.

Only the one who has become free of himself can teach his neighbor in the right way, in accordance with the eternal law of God, guiding, helping and serving him.

If a person would first explore his inner life and recognize and develop his true being, then the spiritual heritage, which God breathed into his spirit body, would come alive through the power of selfless love. Then there would be peace and harmony in this world, and selflessness.

The one who no longer looks to himself, who has conquered himself, can draw from his innermost being, from his eternal being, which is selfless, and bring peace to this world.

The one who has become free of himself emanates love, peace and good will, regardless of what his neighbor thinks and speaks, of what his convictions may be, of what facial expressions and gestures his neighbor displays.

He is not touched by any of this. He recognizes and sees it, but he is above human emotions and inclinations, since none of the same or like nature is present in him.

Another example: If you see the good and beautiful in your neighbor, if his surroundings are pleasant, if his nature is loving and kind and you envy these spiritual qualities, then you have to ask yourself: Have I already worked on acquiring these qualities?

You know that you have not worked on acquiring the qualities of your neighbor, because you face him with envy. If you now strive to emulate him, if you view him as your model, if you want to copy his nature, his characteristics, which means that you want to acquire them on the outside, then you tie yourself to your neighbor, to his qualities.

If you endeavor more and more to come into contact with your neighbor, because you enjoy being near him, because he has what you do not have, but would like to have, if you continue to emulate him, that is, copy him, on the outside, then you are drawing from your neighbor's life force, all in accordance with the intensity of your wanting and your eagerness.

If your neighbor allows himself to be drawn into the same or similar conversations and debates again and again about the things which you, in the end, do not have but want, you draw the life force from your neighbor, your partner in conversation.

These could be conversations about problems or other difficulties, conversations about topics which preoccupy you, about the things you would like to have. First, you have to work spiritually for these things, by actualizing the eternal law, which ultimately puts in order and supplies you with what you need externally in this world as a human being.

By copying all those things which radiated from your neighbor, you cling to him and try again and again to engage him in conversation about things and circumstances which you admire about him, but do not have yourself.

The result is a constant rehashing of the same problems without any change. If the conversation circles around the same topic again and again, then you have an expectation; you want to acquire the things you do not have.

The conversations, which may become hot debates and a clashing of words, show that you do not want to take charge of your life by actualizing the eternal laws. You want to acquire externally what your neighbor has worked for spiritually.

It is also possible that you condemn what you do not have yourself. You condemn what you would like to have.

The person who condemns, condemns only himself. The person who judges his neighbor judges himself. Therefore, recognize the traces of envy and resentment within you.

If you imitate others, then experience who you are first and become aware that you are a child of God which has everything in its soul, the fullness.

Develop the spiritual consciousness, the fullness, and then the fullness will also become externally visible for you. It will supply you with what you need, and beyond that.

And so, develop the positive powers in yourself, the beauty of your inner being, the tenderness of your nature, the warmth, hope, love and confidence.

Awaken within yourself all the aspects which you admire in your neighbor, which are pleasant and which you want to acquire, by actualizing the eternal law, God.

Never emulate your neighbor, but awaken your own ideal, by actualizing and fulfilling the inner life. So awaken it within yourself.

All positive powers are in you; the fullness is in you.

And so, cause your inner being to shine, by ennobling your sensations, thoughts, words and deeds, then you will again become what you truly are: beautiful, noble, free, pure and powerful.

A being that is filled through and through with light will never look at its neighbor enviously, for it has everything it needs, in its inner being as well as externally. Recognize that you have everything in yourself: youth, beauty, grace and loveliness.

You are what you think and feel. You are a body of thought. You are the sum of your thoughts.

The one who has a glowing, youthful, purified soul will not age. He will fade like a leaf on a tree which has unfolded its full splendor in the summertime.

To fade is not to age. Like a leaf on a tree, your physical body fades, because it is a nature body, which belongs to this earth. Within it is the becoming and the passing away, the law of matter.

The tree of life in man is the spirit. The one who looks carefully at the branches of a tree recognizes that even in fall it already prepares for spring. It is similar with a person who is filled with light. He fades, but does not age.

The inner being, the spring of the soul, the purity of the inner being, radiates throughout the outer shell; it buds anew.

In the process of fading, youth already shimmers through again, the spirituality of the inner being, the light-filled soul. It is the grace and loveliness and the fundamental principle of life which God has placed into his being: love, peace and harmony, all in all, the divine selflessness. And so, recognize the ideal within yourself. See it as real before you!

Know that you are perfect and strive for this perfect ideal, the perfect being in you, by ennobling your thoughts, not by thinking negatively about your neighbor, but by recognizing the good in all things, affirming it and thus feeling and thinking kindly.

The one who strives daily to see the good in all things, regardless of external appearances, will gradually bring out the spiritual aspects which God breathed into him: love, harmony and peace.

These divine aspects of your soul are your very basic, original nature, which is your spiritual mentality: either the divine mentality of Wisdom or of Patience, of Order or of Will, depending on what you predominantly bear within you as divine heritage. This is what molds your true nature.

All of the divine natures and characteristics of God bear within love, beauty, gracefulness, loveliness and divine selflessness. Therefore, do not emulate a different ideal. Restrain your envy and develop your own nature within you.

And so, what the person himself feels, thinks and says is what he is. When you live selflessly, when you live from within to without, when you live close to God, you live consciously. Then you will never judge and reject your neighbor; you will never think and speak negatively about him, because these aspects of the human ego are no longer present in you.

You have become selfless and therefore you are above the human stirrings and inclinations of your fellow man. He does not upset you anymore, because the same or similar qualities are no longer present in you since you no longer expect anything. You have everything you need, and beyond that.

When a person has matured spiritually, his correspondences will dwindle. The individual will realize this when in his sensations and thoughts he is above the things of this world, the inclinations and stirrings of his fellow man, when his sensations and thoughts are the same as his words: noble, pure and kind.

When a person has only positive feelings, thoughts and words for his neighbor, he has become selfless. He has awakened in himself all the things which he had envied in the past about his neighbor and become irritated about.

And so, the one who has raised his being to the divine in himself thinks and speaks about his neighbor in only a positive way, even though he recognizes the negativities in and on his neighbor.

31

When your being is permeated by God's love, your deeds will be selfless. You will let justice come before right. Justice is divine, right is human.

A man of the spirit, a just person, will tell everyone what is just, according the law of love. He will also give to each what the person needs to live justly, insofar as it is possible for the person to do this and if he sees that his neighbor uses these gifts for the benefit of his soul.

The one who demands his rights wants to gain something for himself. And so, he is egotistical, because he wants to maintain and keep his right. But whatever a person wants to hold onto because it is his right, he will lose.

The truly wise man does not insist on his rightness; he is just. He talks in accordance with the law and acts according to the eternal love.

But the one who demands his rights shows in turn who he is. He reveals his base world of feelings and thoughts, his egotism, also called selfishness.

People who insist on their rightness think only of themselves. They want to preserve their base ego. The one who disputes with his neighbor disputes with God.

God is just! God does not dispute with His child. He gives it as much as it can bear and use in the right way.

The one who disputes with his neighbor disputes with God, thus burdening his soul. For every sensation, every thought, every word as well as every deed are registered by the soul. The positive powers imbue soul and man with light and spirit.

Negative sensations, thoughts, words and deeds burden the soul. They fill soul and man with shadow. The result of all the negativities is then harshness, unkindness, brutality, conflict, destruction and much more.

The positive as well as the negative aspects of man have their effects. The positive aspects bring about peace, harmony, love, secureness, happiness and health. The negative aspects scatter; they press towards wanting to have and to possess more. The person no longer knows himself. He only wants to achieve and reach what matter, the world, offers its own.

The ego-awareness of a person, his base nature, says again and again: I am my own best friend. Through these self-centered thoughts — that is, thoughts focused on himself, on the person — the person imposes limits upon himself.

Through this, his spiritual consciousness becomes so narrow that he finally loves only himself and those people who are inclined towards him and live in his immediate surroundings.

When a person is his own best friend, then everything outside of his immediate surroundings is foreign to him.

His fellow man, who lives outside of his narrow scheme of thought, who is not a part of his surroundings, of his intimate circle, is a stranger to him.

What a worldly person sees that is outside of his consciousness, he belittles; he judges his neighbor, or looks enviously at his fellow man. Often he sees the latter only as a satellite of his ego whom he just barely tolerates, because his fellow man complies with his conceptions and wishes and flatters him, thus aggrandizing him.

The self-centered person — that is, the person caught up in the world — on the one hand rejects his fellow man, because the latter is often not like him and so he avoids him, or, he secretly imitates him out of envy and resentment.

The one who wants to be free from his neighbor's views and opinions, his narrow-minded thoughts, should develop his true ideal, his spiritual being. By actualizing the holy eternal laws, a person finds his way to his higher ideals and values, thus attaining the fulfillment of life. The one who lives in fulfillment has actualized the laws, and they will then serve him.

Therefore, O man, be prepared to develop your true higher self!

Put your thoughts in order and think positively. Become still. Put reins on your tongue. Say only what is necessary. Become noble and kind. If you have learned to think, live and act in accordance with the laws, you will become selfless and a master who has conquered his base ego or masters it anew daily until it has dissolved and the I Am, the divine principle, the heritage which lies within you, becomes apparent. Then you live in fulfillment, because you are filled with the power of love.

The true nature of man is selfless, eternally giving love. And so, your true nature is love, peace and harmony. If these divine aspects are effective in you, you also keep your life in order and the divine Will becomes your will.

People who have conquered themselves are wise, not intellectual. They draw from the divine power, from their developed consciousness. They speak from the truth.

People of the spirit let justice rule over right. They are disciplined and earnest, wherever and whenever earnestness is called for. But the truly enlightened person is also cheerful even in earnestness, because he has found himself.

People of the spirit, who are filled by the love of God, are joyful, peaceful and harmonious. Their inner glow is the radiation of selfless love.

Only a peaceful person can truly be joyful. The one who is peaceful has developed the aspects of divine Patience, Love and Mercy and is thus consciously a son or daughter of God. Thus, a person radiates what he is, human or spiritual.

Therefore, recognize yourself:

What you think and say shows who you are.

*How You Dine
and What You Eat
Shows Who You Are*

Introduction

The following text *"How You Dine and What You Eat Shows Who You Are"* contains the explicit advice that a person should not castigate himself in any way. Every castigation, no matter whether it concerns food, beverages, clothing or anything else has its side effects.

In the long run, the effect of every castigation is discontentment. Very often it triggers envy, quarrel and enmity.

And so, we are not telling you to change your diet overnight. We are not telling you to no longer value higher quality clothing and a gracious home.

Instead, change your attitude and your way of life gradually!

Oppose negative thoughts with noble thoughts!

Forgive your neighbor and ask for forgiveness!

Do not speak ill of your neighbor, do not defame him!

The one who is against his neighbor in thoughts, words and actions is against God because God, the life, is in every human being. The one who is against his neighbor violates the life, the law, God.

First ennoble your way of thinking and speaking!

Make it a habit to see the good in everything!

Realize that the gifts, the food, come from the greatest giver, from God. Express your thankfulness and take it in with reverence before the life. Then your attitude will change, the radiation of your body will become finer and your senses will become purer.

Your diet will also change automatically and you will eat less and less meat and fish until your eating habits change as of themselves. In the course of your inner development, you will gradually let go of strong drinks and turn ever more to nature, which holds everything ready for you.

And do not imitate others in terms of your clothing and the furnishing of your home.

Observe nature, how it adorns itself in spring and summer in honor of the Almighty. It does not question the luxuriant growth and multitude of colors and forms; it lets it happen.

Nor should you refuse the desire for a dress or a beautiful piece of furniture, thinking that the one who strives towards the Eternal does not need these or the like any longer.

And do not imitate your neighbor when he thinks, lives and dresses in a different way than you.

Observe your life, ennoble yourself and you will dress and live and show yourself according to your own nature.

Let nature be an example for you. It radiates in its multitude of harmonious colors and forms to the honor of God.

You should live in a moderate way, not excessively. You should not revel in prosperity and wealth.

However, recognize yourself as a child of God and above all adorn yourself with the virtue and beauty of your own true nature. The one who is beautiful in his inner being, whose radiation is fine, will also express this externally. A pretty dress that corresponds to your nature and a nice home that is fitting to you convey pleasure and create harmony. Colors and shapes stimulate your inner being as well as your outer nature, your mood and your world of thoughts.

A person who is joyful inside will also express this externally, in his clothes and home and in his entire behavior, as well as at the table and in the choice of his food. For how you dine and what you eat shows who you are.

The one who ennobles his soul by raising his thinking, his aspirations and striving to God will not live in want and poverty. God gives to His own as much as is good for their soul.

Therefore, man should be thankful for everything, for joy and sorrow, for health and sickness, for clothing, shelter and food.

The task and the great chance of a life on earth lies in improving the quality of our soul, its degree of illumination, its power of vibration and radiation. Therefore, recognize yourself in the expression of your life.

Become a reformer of your life by ennobling and refining yourself through an alignment with the divine.

Within the dimension of time, you are given the opportunity for a quick spiritual development to higher things, a spiritual evolution. You are still in the temporal.

Use it!

God's mills grind for the good as well as for the sinner.

Gabriele
Würzburg, March 1986

The enlightened person recognizes you

God is love.

God is harmony.

God is the basis of spiritual ethics and morals.

God is omnipresent.

God is life.

God, the life, is all in all things. His power is in everything that lives.

His power is the stream of selfless love.

God is the giver. God gives Himself in everything that is.

You are from God.

You are divine in your origin.

God is absolute love.

Since you are divine, you, too, are love.

The law, God, is love.

In your origin, you, too, are the law.

If a person violates the law, the principle of life, the highest ethics and morals, the selfless love, then he turns away from the Absolute Law, God, the selfless love, and puts himself into the law of cause and effect, into the causal law.

Every burdened soul and every burdened person contribute to making the law of cause and effect, the causal law, come into effect. The sum of the wrong behavior of all people is controlled by the causal law of the world. This influences an individual according to his former and present world of thoughts.

The effectiveness of the causal law is formed by energies transformed down from the Absolute Law, God, which is selfless love.

High ethics and morals mold the character, the nature, of a spiritual person

He will think nobly, speak selflessly, act kindly and his nature is sovereign. He stands above human stirrings and inclinations, also above the pretentious behavior of his neighbor, above his opinions and conceptions. His conduct is harmonious and balanced; his body is upright, his look clear. The person is flexible and young, despite the years during which he fades.

Further principles of highest ethics and morals are wisdom and kindness. People with these principles of life are active and constructive, supportive and serving; they are patient, merciful and orderly. What they do, they do completely. What they promise, they keep. They are punctual, sacrificing, benevolent, patient, loving, gentle, humble and reliable in all things.

Souls and human beings who, because of their offenses against the divine law, have fallen into the law of cause and effect get more and more entangled in selfishness which is the opposite pole of selfless love. This happens unless the person recognizes in time his filiation in God.

According to his soul burden, the self-centered person thinks only of himself and relates everything that exists to himself.

Because he is self-centered, the person caught up by the world relates everything that his neighbor says about him, the positive as well as the negative, to himself.

Through this, the person merges with the temporal, with matter, more and more. He becomes insatiable and ever more focused on himself.

Through his egocentricity, a person creates new patterns of thought, for example, that his neighbor has to think and live in the same way he does, or that his neighbor should not have more nor less than he himself has.

Through these thought patterns, ever more knots are made by the individual which lead to karmic ties by which human beings are bound to one another. In this or in future lives, they are then led together to clear up the cause that was once set.

The one who is not well disposed toward his neighbor or constantly rebukes him and speaks negatively about him, thus creating causes which harm his neighbor or cause him pain, is bound to this person. He can find liberation only when the other person forgives him. This is what then brings about the release of the karmic tie.

In this way, a stubborn person who is not aligned with the law of life adds onto his own fate day by day, a fate that is the sum of all his wrongdoing. The different blows of fate which hit people and take place in this world are based on former causes that have become effective.

People who have not concerned themselves with the law of sowing and reaping think that a blow of fate happens by chance. Such people can make the fate of their neighbor their own, by anxiously brooding about whether they, too, will have to suffer the same or a similar fate.

The one who is daily anxious about whether the same or a similar fate as his neighbor's could happen to himself very often creates a cause based on his anxiety and brooding, the result of which he fears.

This anxious thinking can cause the fate of his neighbor or a similar fate, which at first did not lie in him, to build up in him, in his soul.

Thoughts are forces that become effective in and upon a person. They become thought forms which influence the body and, depending on their intensity, change its structure and mass. Light-filled thoughts imbue soul and person with light. Dark thoughts darken the soul and mark the shell, the person, accordingly.

The light-filled person is a spiritual person who radiates the spiritual ethics and morals as a characteristic, as something that has grown within him: in the shape of his body, in the posture of his body, in his movements, facial expressions, in his thoughts and words, at the table and in his choice of foods.

In the expression of how he eats and what he eats, a person reveals who he is.

The one who ignores the causal law and indulges in his life on earth without restraint indirectly separates himself more and more from God, the Absolute Law.

The more a person gets entangled with his ego, that is, the greater his egotism is, the more knots develop for him in the law of sowing and reaping. Because of a self-centered way of thinking and living, that is, because of the desire to possess, to be and to have, a continuously growing gulf develops between God and the person.

God is All-harmony

If the thinking, feeling and wanting of a person is mainly focused on himself, if he is only interested in going after external, material things, if he strives to train his intellect in order to be someone important in the world, in order to strengthen his ego, to add to his possessions, to fulfill his desires and push through his opinions, then he moves more and more away from the All-harmony, God, the Absolute Law that is love.

Through this, he falls more and more into the law of cause and effect. This law shows him his unlawful behavior, which eventually results in blows of fate. At the proper time, when the corresponding planet-radiation irradiates the field of fate in the soul, it comes into effect.

The time in which the cause reaches its effect is determined by the corresponding planetary irradiation under which the person comes when creating cause after cause because of a wrong way of thinking and living.

God, the All-harmony, is a predetermined eternal rhythm, it is symphony and sound

The whole pure Being sings in honor of God. It is the universal rhythm, the harmonious melodious sound, the universal orchestra.

When man moves away from the divine rhythm of eternal perfect love, from the All-harmony, then disharmony and mental disturbances move in. His soul and body rhythm become edgy and awkward; his nature becomes undisciplined towards his neighbor and himself.

The undisciplined behavior of a self-centered person becomes noticeable in all life situations, and thus in the way he takes in food, too.

And so, how he dines and what and how he eats show who he really is: what the make-up of his soul is, which burdens the soul exhibits, whether it lives in the all-harmonious rhythm, in God, or is captured by the dissonances of this world.

The more world-oriented, that is, the more human, the individual has become, the more he has indulged in the world of sensual pleasures with his desires and longings, the more passionate he is.

To the passionate person, nothing that surrounds him and that he can get hold of is holy. He sees only his own interests and wants to have everything for himself. Persons who think only of themselves and who live only for themselves try to draw to themselves everything that they can get hold of.

The one who lives in egotism, who is selfish, binds in turn other people to him. They should be his slaves, without a will of their own.

Such strong-willed people who are only concerned about themselves also tend to make their second neighbors, the animals and plants, slaves of their ego. They kill and rob nature, thus deliberately violating the world of nature for their own sake alone.

The one who thinks only of himself does not recognize that in the end he has become a slave to his own desires and passions.

The desires and passions become stronger to the degree the person clouds himself with them by having the same thoughts and desires over and over again. In the same measure that he intensifies these with the same or similar thoughts and words, they also become effective in and through him — visible for those who are on a higher spiritual level.

Desires and passions also form fog-like shapes — just as every thought that keeps returning becomes a fog-like shape.

Desires and passions, the vibrating, fog-like thought formations that are invisible to most of us, influence in turn the self-centered person. They inspire him and lead him deeper and deeper into the world of selfishness, into his own slavery.

An egotistical and greedy person who strives only to satisfy his own desires and longings is a self-centered, angry, hectic person who has become distant from the All-harmony, God.

And so, the person who is self-centered is selfish. He lives in wishful thinking and wanting, in self-love.

Very often such people can no longer distinguish between selfless love and selfish love — until they experience on themselves what selfish love and selfless love is. Fate knows the path of recognition for every blind person.

The law, God, is highest ethics and morals.

People who strive for the absolute life, who long for the highest ethics and morals, will be able to establish without effort the spiritual ethics, a life in and with the Spirit, basing themselves upon the basic principles of the ethics and morals of earth.

Those who strive for high ethics and morals are natural people, whose inner maturity is expressed in all situations of life, including in the way they take in their food: How a person dines and what he eats shows who he is.

The inner as well as the outer ethics and morals, which are the basic rules of behavior on earth, are innate to the spiritual person. People whose spiritual consciousness grows more and more into the divine live according to the basic law of love. They are harmonious, balanced people with naturalness and a spiritual aura. This is the expression of inner maturity.

People whose true nature is spirituality, an attribute of their being, are mostly independent people who have not fallen under the imitative drive of the masses. In their thoughts and sensations, in their desires, they are not dependent on their neighbor. They do not want what their neighbor has acquired with effort; they do not want anything of the same or like kind. They are free in their thinking and living.

They are the so-called spiritual free-thinkers who recognize the spiritual life as the true life. They personify the principles of highest ethics and morals in every sphere of their life. Their way of thinking and living also marks their table manners. They dine the way they think. They also choose what they eat accordingly.

People who are striving for the actualization of the spiritual principles of life, for the highest ideals and values, draw from the true source, from the selfless love which fulfills them and sets them free.

The one who tries to lead a life that is selfless, pure in morals and deeds, gradually finds his way to the kingdom of All-harmony, to God, of which Jesus said: "My kingdom is not of this world."

By the effort to become selfless, the spiritual person finds his way into the kingdom of the inner being, the divine universal rhythm which is the highest symphony and sound, and thus music.

The fullness from God,
the universal pure life,
is the highest symphony

The All-harmony that is reflected in the naturalness and freedom of a spiritual person who resembles the image, the divine, has the effect of countless suns on many people. Invisibly, but perceivable for many who are spiritually awakened, such people radiate the highest ethics and morals, the purity of the heavens, the light-filled soul which dwells in the person, the Kingdom of God in man.

People of the spirit respect and cherish life. They recognize the essence of all forms of life as a part of their own life. They cherish and love the nature kingdoms and thank their Creator for everything that the earth, nature, gives from its fullness.

Every person bears witness of himself. He need not open his mouth. His traits, his character, mark his external look. His whole appearance tells who he is.

A person also shows who he is by the way he takes in his meals. For the way he dines and what he eats shows his character, his true nature. The deeper the soul of a person has fallen, the darker his radiation, the more disharmonious is that person.

The human body
is the condensed radiation of the soul

The positive and negative aspects of the soul mark and shape the body.

The noble and pure aspects of the soul as well as the impure, cruel egocentricity of a person become visible externally, in and on the body. Therefore, figuratively speaking, the body is his soul, that is, the expression of what is active in the soul and not of what lies in it.

It can be that what is still latent in the soul – the positive as well as the negative aspects – may not come into effect until years or decades later or even in a further life, either in the soul realms or in another human life.

Therefore, a young person with a young body, an attractive person, does not necessarily have a pure soul: Just as nature adorns itself in spring, in the same way the physical body shows itself – whether the soul is pure or whether the impure has not yet come into effect.

Spring adorns itself with colors and forms; it clothes the earth in a beautiful, balanced, even magnificent dress. In summer nature shows itself in its full splendor. In autumn it brings out the ripeness of the fruit that it had displayed as blooming splendor in spring. Winter brings poverty. Trees and bushes are bare. The season is cold, icy and frosty. The days are shorter, nights are longer. The sun shines its warm rays onto another part of the earth that is now more turned towards it.

A human life is also like this image, that is, a human life can be compared to nature.

How quickly the bright and clear weather can change in human existence! The attractive form of the body can be seized by winter within a short time; a cold and frosty disposition brings forth its fruits. The inner aspects that are at the point of coming into effect mark the mind of the person, be he young or old.

In this way a young, attractive body can change shape very rapidly and be marked by grief and sickness by what was present in the soul and which came into effect according to the law of cause and effect, the causal law.

People who are in the full maturity of their life and have had to suffer little grief, whose features are even and beautiful, whose surroundings are harmonious, who have everything they need to embellish their lives anew daily, will also be seized by fate if a burden is present in their soul that has to come into effect because of the causes which were set earlier. In a life full of sunshine, confidence and hope for the material, a blow of fate can suddenly overshadow and darken everything.

And so, what was still lying latent in the soul came into effect and seized the person. This shows that from one day to the next a person can lose all his property and possessions which he acquired with effort. What remains can be a disappointed person whose resignation wrinkles his once beautiful and even features, aging his body within a short period.

Another person, in turn, goes through the four seasons of his life on earth unperturbed. He has property and possessions; he is rich, respected and healthy. His appearance is pleasant to the people of the world; his behavior, as far as he can see, is impeccable.

But the spiritual person, the enlightened one, looks deeper. He recognizes that the apparently impeccable and very often irreproachable behavior that is shaped by the intellect is only acquired and did not grow from within.

The purely intellectual person, who is dominated by his mind, does not have the intelligence, that is, the strength of an opened consciousness. The divine intelligence, the logos that knows about all things and that raises man to true wisdom and to high ethics and morals, to selfless life, is still covered up in him to a great extent.

The one person is seized by fate, the cause that was latent until now and that comes into effect in this life. The other one seemingly lives a carefree life, untouched by the causes which perhaps still lie dormant in his soul.

So despite a shadowed soul, a human being can have everything he has wished for in this life; he can satisfy all his desires, thus believing that all good spirits are on his side. In the behavior and life of a fellow man who is marked by worldly things, the wise one recognizes very well the faults and weaknesses which his fellow man has not yet recognized himself.

Although his life on earth does not show the burden yet and although his soul is still attached to this world and is not yet touched by its own fate, he is nevertheless already marked by his behavior. And so, the burden that is present in the soul and the burden that will still be added during this life are in this case still latent.

The person who does not presently recognize the effects of the causes that are still latent in his soul can nevertheless make of this life on earth a gain for his spiritual development, by living and acting according to the law of selfless love. The good that he actualizes and fulfills radiates back into his soul as light and can illuminate many a shadow still hidden in the depths of his soul and dissolve them in part or wholly.

Then this person will not have to then bear and experience in full measure the effects that come up later.

People who are still with this world and are subject to the opinions and conceptions of their fellow man — who themselves are still very self-centered — look only at the outer appearance of their fellow man, at the shell as it shows itself, but is not.

Therefore, the people of this world look at things superficially. They see only the external vibration-form and very often let themselves be deluded and led astray by this.

An enlightened person does not see a person merely in the way he shows himself. He looks much deeper. He looks at the effects of the thoughts on the body, because the person is molded by his thoughts and ways of acting. His nutrition, what he eats and how he dines are also reflected on the body. His behavior, gestures and facial expressions, his choice of food and movements, as well as the way he takes in his food show who he is.

A truly enlightened person looks into the depths of his fellow man, behind the mask of his conduct and bearing and sees the characteristics as they really are, not as they seem to be. He also sees the pure in the person as well as the impure.

Everybody shows who he is,
whether he is aware of this or not

To the truly enlightened person, his neighbor is not unknown, not even when he sees him for the first time. A truly enlightened person sees his fellow man in the depths of the latter's consciousness. He recognizes what is lying there and what is light, but he can also see the dark and disturbing influences that affect the other one.

The words of a person show who he is. His demeanor, his behavior, his clothes and his home show who he is. The shape of his body is also an expression of his soul.

The enlightened one looks into everything, into every word, every gesture and facial expression, into the conduct of his fellow man. The play of expressions also discloses the inner state of a person.

The body is the expression of the soul. Soul and body, in turn, influence their own surroundings. The external quality of the life of a person, the way he shows himself, the food he prefers, the way he eats show who and what he is.

Your hairstyle and your clothes show who you are. The spiritual development is also expressed in the clothing of a person and in his immediate surroundings, in his home, which, in turn, reflects his inner state.

In this booklet I mainly want to point out the features and characteristics of people which also become manifest in the way they take in food. A person chooses his kind of nourishment on the basis of his spiritual and material orientation. What he eats and how he eats shows who he is.

A spiritually oriented person will never castigate himself. In order to find his way to the highest ethics and morals, he will first put his thoughts into order and see the positive aspects in everything, even in the apparently negative. He will strive to see his neighbor as his brother and to be well-disposed towards him. In all forms of life, in animals as well as in plants, he will recognize the spiritual life that maintains everything that lives.

By doing this his senses will turn inward. The nobility of his soul begins to bud and to grow. This way of life, through a positive orientation of thoughts and feelings, has the effect that the person switches from coarse foods like meat and fish to the gifts that nature gives him. He will not make this change from one day to the next, but will do it gradually.

In order to remain or become healthy and harmonious, it is not the external change in nutrition that is important, but one's thoughts have to be ennobled so that the person can become what he is: a spiritual being in the earthly garment.

Because of the readjustment of his thoughts towards a selfless way of feeling, thinking and speaking, the person will also take up an upright, respectful posture at the table, before the gifts that he has received from God, his Lord, for the strengthening of his body and his soul. As his thoughts become light and harmonious, the person will be lent wings by the harmonious cosmic energies.

The effect is that in the course of this transformation, the dull, materialistic and uncontrolled person will become a harmoniously thinking human being, whose body will be more and more thoroughly radiated by spiritual power, thereby showing inner lightness and flexibility. This in turn results in a preference for a lighter diet that he will prepare in a mild way, avoiding the pungency of salt and hot spices more and more.

The harder a person is in his way of thinking and living, in treating his fellow man ruthlessly, the coarser, spicier and heavier is his food. The lighter his thoughts, the more buoyant, harmonious and spiritually dynamic a person is, the lighter his nutrition is.

He avoids a lot of salt and hot spices. He will reduce alcohol and nicotine more and more and finally have but a glass of wine when he is in the company of loving and sociable people. He will not crave it; instead, without being driven, he will take the wine, the alcoholic beverage, moderately, according to the basic rules of spiritual ethics and morals.

I repeat: People of the spirit whose consciousness rests in the divine are people who have turned within, who have become internalized. The measure for the internalization of a person does not lie in a frantic effort to give a spiritual impression, by showing himself as he is not through external concentration and effort of will.

A person's mask, the way he shows himself externally, does not always present his true characteristics. Very often it is acquired or put on. Generally speaking, it is the illusion with which he deceives those like him.

The life of a person can be very many-layered. It is marked by different features, depending on the way he expresses them in his thinking and speaking. In his behavior he shows who he is. He remains bound to his human inclinations, to his personal ego, until he begins to strive towards higher ideals and values.

With his mask, the person wants to hide his unevenness and ugliness from this world. And so, he wants to conceal what he really is.

What a person thinks, that is what he is and not what he says. People of this world are like actors on the stage of the world. In some cases, the person plays his role very well. He is so absorbed in his role that he finally believes he is what he pretends to be. In reality, he represses his human impulses in many situations, thus making of himself a slave and an actor.

Through the roles that people play on the stage of the world, they achieve many a thing. Day after day they make a new entrance. Despite the applause they receive from their like, they remain dissatisfied and unhappy in many cases.

For every actor there comes a time when he falls out of his role and reveals to those who have applauded him thus far who he really is.

People who speak from their masks, the so-called actors who cover up their feelings and thoughts, are disguised only to those like them. But for the truly seeing, every person remains an open book.

The body of thoughts, the radiation of a person, is what he truly is. The spiritually perceiving have learned to comprehend the structure of thoughts of the individual, not what he speaks, not what he pretends to be in words, gestures and appearance.

The body of thoughts is what a person actually is, not what he pretends to be. It is the thought-body that shows who he is.

However disciplined or externally concentrated a person may be, for the spiritual person he is an open book. Nothing is hidden to the pure person. But to the impure one, everything is hidden, because he looks only at the shell and not at the core which is the essential.

To the pure person everything is evident, to the impure person everything is hidden. What the worldly person cannot see he dismisses by saying: God does not let us look into His mysteries.

God has no mysteries to the one who is with Him. However, the one who violates God's laws draws the veil of ignorance over divine wisdom and merely looks at other masks through his own mask.

Everything is evident to the truly enlightened one. The one who is open for God, for His laws, can also see the law and the law shows him what is truth and what is appearance.

The one who trains himself spiritually by way of recognition and actualization, the one who really makes efforts to recognize himself, the one who applies inner and outer discipline and concentration, is the one who takes the first steps on the path to spiritualization.

External discipline and external concentration alone are not the signs of a truly wise person. The inner attitude towards all people and things is a true inner discipline and deep concentration.

The truly wise person lives consciously. His nature is cheerful, balanced, noble and perfect. He lives from within, from his opened consciousness. The naturalness of the pure soul, the high nobility and the morals which are the highest virtues of life, the selfless love, can be seen in his entire behavior.

The "personalness" of a person is his self-centeredness; it is the body of thought that marks the person. The personality wants to display something to the world.

The impersonal life is not a display, but intelligence

People of the world who promote their personality make frantic efforts to maintain their ego and to preserve, support and expand it with the help of a trained intellect.

Personal strivings are intellectual strivings. They have nothing in common with the true intelligence, the logos, God, the opened divine consciousness.

The intellect is acquired. It also includes thought forms that surround the intellectual as satellites and influence him when he thinks and speaks according to these vibrating complexes.

Like always attracts like and they stimulate one another mutually. People of the spirit are led by the logos, the highest consciousness. But people of the world are led by the world, by the thought forms that surround them.

And so people who live with the world, whose intellectual aspirations are entirely oriented towards the world, are inspired by their own thought forms which they have created and go on creating through their human, self-centered thinking.

Every thought that is not lawful, that is, that diverges from the law of God, remains effective within and around the person.

Thought forms accompany the person. They are with him as companions, so to speak, insofar as his thoughts circle around his own person. It is essential to distinguish between intellect and intelligence. The intellect is not divine wisdom. The intellect is learned and acquired knowledge, something that has been put on and did not grow from the consciousness, God, but, as mentioned before, was learned.

The divine intelligence is the logos, the consciousness of the soul, the law, God. The purer the soul is, the more all-encompassing the consciousness, God, the divine intelligence, comes forth, inspiring the person and leading him to true greatness and inner wisdom.

And so, the divine intelligence
in man is the divine logos
that knows of all things,
that is all in all things

The divine intelligence in a person, the opened consciousness of his soul, does not need an external mask.

The person who lives in the consciousness of God does not need to strive for knowledge. He knows, because he has found the truth; he has found his divine nature.

The one who has come closer to his divine nature by means of a conscious life that is aligned with the highest intelligence, by the actualization of the holy laws, has little intellect, but he does have the highest wisdom. And so, he is in the perfection of his life.

People of the spirit who are in the perfection of their lives will also externally personify the love and wisdom of God. They are not subject to human compulsions, because they personify the attributes of a selfless life in thoughts, words and deeds. They are uncomplicated people who, within moments, grasp a situation and put it in the proper perspective. In the world, at their place of work, they accomplish their tasks to the best of their abilities, calmly, consciously, purposefully and with concentration.

The life of a spiritual person is harmony. His movements and gestures, his entire behavior, his smile, his graceful nature — the world calls it charm — are the movements of the pure soul within the person, which is close to the goal of the divine Being, the All-harmony.

People of the spirit are purposeful.
Whatever they do, they fulfill in harmony

People of the spirit are not indolent or boring, but rather active since God is dynamism. And so, they are dynamic, active people who live, think and work consciously, from within harmony.

The thoughts of a person mark his body. His way of thinking and speaking, the way he eats and the kind of food he takes in, the clothes he wears and the furnishing of his home reflect the degree of purity of his soul.

As revealed before, people of the spirit are people with divine attributes; they are dynamic, joyful people who are independent of the opinions and desires of their neighbor or of his life habits.

People who strive for perfection live from within. Their feelings and thoughts are their words. Their words correspond to their feelings and thoughts.

Every person — the one who thinks positively as well as the one who thinks negatively — shows in his outer appearance who he is. His behavior shapes and marks his earthly garment, his body.

People of the spirit, whose thoughts and words are noble, live in the totality of creation. They are nature loving since they recognize the Creator of all Being in all life forms. They bring Him their love by selflessly loving whatever lives: animals, plants, stones. To them all life is also their life.

Through this, they have consciously become creation-thoughts, since their thoughts and senses are linked with the All-harmony.

In this way, creation lives consciously through them and they are one with all things and all beings, with all Being.

The whole universe is the law, God.

The law, God, is sound, melody.
It is the All-harmony, God

The stars as well as the minerals, flowers, grasses and animals, all life forms, are consciousness. Thus, everything that lives is consciousness.

The consciousness is melody. The sound of the individual species of life corresponds to the state of consciousness of the life forms.

The pure Being, the spiritual universe, is the fullness. The pure spirit beings live in this fullness. They do not strive for possessions and wealth; they have everything that was created by God. Everything that is pure lives in this fullness.

The essence of all Being is effective in the spirit being. It draws from this essence and lives with it. And so, it lives in and with God, the fullness.

Everything is sound,
everything is symphony

The spiritual universe is like an orchestra. It is called the All-harmony, God. Countless degrees and spheres of consciousness come together in the one sound that is called the All-harmony. In this way, the All-harmony is the heavenly music of the spheres.

Every form of life has its sound, that is, every form of consciousness is a little symphony in the All-harmony, which is sound, symphony and orchestra at the same time.

Everything is vibration. Every vibration has its tone. The soul as well as the physical body, the person, are vibrating bodies of sound that vibrate and sound according to the development of their spirit consciousness.

Person and soul have their sound according to the burden of the soul and the habits of the person.

The human being is either surrounded by dissonances or by harmonious sounds, depending on his way of thinking and acting. He is the melody which, in the final analysis, he himself plays in his sensations, thoughts, word actions.

Thus, the aspects of consciousness in man are sound. Everything vibrates and produces sound, not audible to the human ear, yet perceivable.

An individual himself shows the way he vibrates. In every gesture, in his way of thinking, living and acting, he shows who he is. All of this forms a musical composition.

Every movement, the way he eats and what, gives evidence of how he vibrates and thus, of how he sounds.

A person can personify the symphonies of the divine, if he thinks and lives divinely. Or he can personify the dissonant tones of the world, if he is oriented to the world, if his thinking, feeling and striving are attached to the things of the earth.

And so, the way a person thinks and lives is how he sounds

His melodies either contribute to raising many people if he is on his path to the divine nature, or he poisons his surroundings if his melody is attuned to the clamor of this world which takes its toll according to the world-ego.

The atmosphere of the earth bears within it a layer of the atmospheric chronicle which is called the world-ego. This is where everything negative, which has been thought and accomplished by human beings throughout all the ages, is stored.

The individual components of this world-ego dissolve only when the concerned soul or person who entered his negativities into the world-ego has atoned and been forgiven or when he has overcome his ego by turning to the divine.

Positive forces are also effective in the atmospheric chronicle, the thinking and living of the true mystics, prophets and enlightened people of all ages.

The positive as well as the negative in the atmospheric chronicle have an effect, in turn, on the people who live in these fields of vibration and are open to these influences through their self-will and imitation of others.

Because of his negative sounds and dissonances man contributes to the decline of the world.

The maturity of a person, his spiritual development towards the divine, shows what level of consciousness he is on and who he is. A person is symphony or dissonance according to how he thinks and lives and how he shows himself.

People who are approaching the All-harmony, God, whose consciousness has progressed, that is, expanded, enough so that they can be led directly by the divine power are uncomplicated, cheerful, natural people with a high degree of intelligence. Their thinking is uncomplicated. They have a quick faculty of perception and the ability to react rapidly.

Their way of thinking and living, their manners and customs also become evident in the way they eat. They will choose and partake of their food according to the nobility, that is, purity, of their souls.

The posture of a spiritually awakened person is upright, just as his character is impeccable and without fault. His life is straightforward. He keeps the spiritual laws and the ones of the earth, insofar as these can be brought into accordance with the divine laws.

Since the spiritual essence, the basis of life, exists in all life forms, truly spiritual people will take in their food in an upright position, knowing that every gift is a gift of God to man. While eating, they will handle fork and knife just as they are themselves: flexibly, harmoniously and calmly.

People of the spirit who are free of external conceptions, opinions and complexes know how to skillfully integrate themselves into the principles found on earth, into the ethical principles of a human perspective. They can bring the inner ethics and morals, which are their nature and disposition, into connection with the human principles of ethics and morals, so that despite everything in the world they remain people of the spirit, who, in the awareness of their strength, are far superior to the worldly man. In their spirituality, they seem to melodically underscore the external ethics with inner harmony, with spiritual ethics and morals, thus showing who they are.

People of the spirit do not gulp down the gifts of God, their food. They will take bite after bite into their mouth, chewing every bite harmoniously and then sending it to the digestive organ in a well-chewed state. They will not shove further bites into a full mouth, but will first swallow one bite before taking another gift onto the spoon or fork, in order to put it into mouth and body.

They will also show themselves externally just as they are in their inner being which is spiritually aligned. If the food is taken in consciously, calmly and harmoniously, then the meal will also be a harmonious sound that touches all those who participate in the meal, stimulating them to even greater harmony.

Since everything is sound, the partaking of food is also sound, and thus a melody

According to his state of consciousness, the individual will eat and thus give out the sounds and resonances that he places into the ingestion of his food.

Just as the entire picture, the whole appearance of a person is, so is the sound of his consciousness, the melody of his soul. Just as he thinks and lives, so does he choose his food and eat it.

People with high ideals and values, who recognize the divine force in everything, will partake of their food in reverence towards God, the giver. They will not gulp down the gifts of God and speak with a full mouth, nor will they drink while their mouth is still full.

People of the spirit are moderate in everything, including food. They are neither demanding nor choosy. They are thankful for the food and take what is offered to them. They know that negative thoughts poison the body more than animal products.

They will not prefer the products of animals, meat and fish in particular, since they know that animals have to give up their life for this.

When spiritual people are the guests of their fellow man and meat and fish is offered to them, they will not indignantly reject the prepared gifts. In this case, too, they know how to keep spiritual and human principles. They will honor and respect the manners and customs of their fellow man to the extent that they can bring these into harmony with their inner attitude. Thus, they will not reject the food. They appreciate the love and expenditure of time from their host. And they will express this by thankfully accepting the food.

People of the spirit who are actualizing spiritual ethics and morals are very sensitive, flexible and tolerant people. They will take from the meat and fish dishes only as much as their inner being can bear and as can be brought into conformity with the spiritual laws of love and peace. As guests at a meal, people of the spirit will not reject the meat and fish offered to them, nor will they consume them with contempt. They will partake of these gifts knowing that they were prepared by loving hands, by the host or hostess who has placed all their skill in it. They will also partake of these gifts harmoniously and thankfully, like any other dish which they can accept according to their inner attitude and maturity.

But the basis for every meal is the gratitude to God for His Creator-power which gives itself to people in the form of condensed substance, as food for soul and body. They will always pray consciously before and after the meal and lift their heart to God to thank Him for everything that He, the all-power, has given them.

People whose spiritual ethics and morals are a basic feature of their inner being will never sit at the table unwashed, unshaven, dressed in dirty, ragged or worn-out clothes.

The table manners of spiritually awakened people are proper, but not exaggerated

Everyone who sits at the table to take a meal has a napkin, a plate, cutlery and a glass if drinks are offered. In one's own home, in the family, a tablecloth should be a matter of course. And a burning candle should not be missing. This outer light is a token of the inner light that stimulates all growth, that brings forth fruit and lets it ripen.

In many cases, the inner ethics and morals can be brought into harmony with the manners of people, insofar as the habits do not culminate in luxuries or a dissolute life, and the person does not indulge in a life of pleasure.

A worldly person can disguise himself only in front of those like him, showing himself as he would like to be seen, but is not in his true nature.

People who live and draw from their inner being, from their true being, can see very well what has grown from within their neighbor and what is only a masquerade. In the conduct of their neighbor, in his movements, they see how he really is. The entire human image, the facial expressions and the way of speaking make clear what sort of spirit rules the person.

Only the one who still wears a mask himself looks at the mask of his fellow man. The one who is still under the pressure of his ego can be deceived by his like, but not the truly wise one who is free of the compulsion to imitate, of wanting to be like this or that person or like the majority of people.

Man as the conscious image of the divine intelligence, which is the embodiment of all beauty, purity, selflessness and nobility, shows himself to the world as he is, irreproachable and conscious.

Such people are usually misunderstood by their fellow man, because they do not make a lot of themselves. Why should they? They have everything they need and more. They are rich because they are peaceful and have made God the center of their lives.

The nobility of the soul comes from a pure and free soul. It shows itself as sound, as a symphony in the gestures and facial expressions of the person. Every conduct shows the nobility of the soul. This also applies to table manners, to a spiritual and noble behavior while partaking of food.

How a person dines and what he eats shows who he is. His manner and his behavior can be a chord from the All-harmony, God, or a dissonance from this world.

Like everything else, food is vibration. Every vibration is sound. And so, a person sounds like his way of thinking, speaking and acting; this is the vibration of his body. According to the vibration of his body, he will also choose his food and stimulants.

The activity of the five senses of man corresponds to his body rhythm. The senses of man are feelers or antennas that probe, on the external, material level, everything that he bears in himself as thoughts and desires.

The senses of a person react according to the momentary rhythm of his human body, its vibration. The thoughts stimulate the senses and the senses, in turn, stimulate the thoughts. This results in wishful thinking and in craving foods that are attuned to the momentary consciousness of the person.

The organs of man are also vibration. They communicate to the brain what they want and prefer, informing the brain which substances they need to stay healthy.

A person chooses his food according to his body rhythm, that is, according to his consciousness.

God is eternal primordial sensation. The primordial sensation is the language of the divine beings. They feel, but they do not think. Their sensation is divine; it is the law.

People of the spirit see in the animal their second neighbor

Animals, too, have their world of sensations, according to their development, to their consciousness. Man calls it instinct. Since animals have feelings or, as man says, they perceive and act instinctively, they are able to feel fear and need when people treat them brutally and cruelly.

Material forms are manifested Creator-power. Hence every animal, like every form of life, is manifested creative power, a part of the divine logos.

The one who violates the life forms acts against himself. The soul of every person, called spirit being when it is pure, possesses within itself all forces, all the spheres of consciousness of infinity and the consciousness-aspects of the minerals, plants and animals, too.

Thus, whoever violates the nature kingdoms, whoever does violence to animals, burdens his soul. He does violence to himself and adds to the structure of his own fate.

If a person prefers meat and fish, if his food consists mainly of this, he contributes to the fact that animals are killed to supply meat. This means that he burdens his soul, just as much as those who kill animals for this and other purposes, as with animal experiments, for example.

The spirit body is the law, God. It consists of the essence of all life forms. And so, the body of a spirit being consists of all the energies of consciousness of the minerals, plants, animals, and so on. The essence of the stars is also a part of the spirit body.

Everything that lives is of divine origin, and is thus divine. The divine is life. Life is in man and thus everything that lives exists as essence in man.

The essence of the totality is contained in every soul and in all forms of being

And so, the one who deliberately sins against his second neighbor, the animal, is responsible before God for his egotistical deeds. He sins against God and in this way burdens his soul.

The Lord said: "Whatever you do to the least of My brothers, you have done to Me." This statement also refers to the whole, because everything is spirit of His spirit and power of His power.

The spirit of infinity is the Creator-power that penetrates and maintains all life forms. The Creator-power, God, is also the strength of your brother and your sister.

The spirit being in development is raised to be a child of God by the forces which are effective in the spirit being and in man, and are called the Father-Mother-forces. It is from these forces that the filiation characteristics of Patience, Love and Mercy emerge.

Everything comes from the unity, God, and lives in the unity, God. The unity is the law.

From the divine perspective, all men and beings as well as all forms of life live in unity. And so, whatever man does to his neighbor as well as to his second neighbor, the animals, plants and the minerals, he does to himself, thus burdening his soul.

God is the life.

If man deliberately violates life, no matter which form of life, be it people, animals or plants and minerals, he sins against God.

Everything that lives is the expression of the Creator-power, it is God, it is unity, it is life

Therefore, people of the spirit will not kill as an end to itself. They know that what they do to the least of creatures falls back upon them.

Nature in its diversity offers everything that man needs to live. Nature freely gives man all upbuilding and maintaining substances that he needs for his body to become and to stay healthy.

Man does not become sick because his body lacks this or that trace element or substance. He becomes sick because he thinks, speaks and acts in the wrong way.

Because of this false way of thinking and acting, a person changes his body structure. As a result, the forces of nature cannot be as effective as they are when God gives them to a person so that he may be and remain healthy and strong.

The body that is marked and shaped by false thinking, by large quantities of meat, by cravings, sensuality and all other passions can often no longer properly absorb the substances of nature. Such a body is dispolarized, that is, oriented to external stimuli and substances. Through this, it is no longer possible for many to absorb the necessary substances from the products of nature, substances that benefit the whole maintenance of the body, that strengthen and invigorate it and keep it healthy.

Because of the external stimulation of the senses, the body — which in the last analysis is a nature-body — becomes a body of the senses that craves only external products, meat and fish and all other culinary pleasures.

But the one who knows the eternal laws and fulfills them will receive from the divine multiplicity and love, which flows to each person in manifold ways and means.

Through this, he becomes a noble, modest and selfless person. His nature becomes balanced and harmonious, his behavior spiritual, even noble.

The one who consciously takes in the products of nature as a gift from God to man will see the ruling hand of God in all things, thus finding his way to his inner being where harmony and peace are present.

As a result, such people, whom I call people of the spirit, are radiant and dynamic. Their movements and gestures are graceful; their manners and customs are in accordance with the law of God.

The strivings and aspirations of a spiritual person are irreproachable. He always strives to fulfill the will of God.

The inner life of a person is expressed externally. People who live in the light of the All-harmony, whose way of thinking, feeling and acting is ennobled, personify the spiritual life, the high ethics and morals. In connection with this statement "high ethics and morals," I should like to briefly mention the laws of evolution, which are lived through, or when necessary suffered through, by many spiritually awakened people, so that they may reach the highest goal, the union with the divine in man.

The one who lives in God knows about his divineness, about his existence as a divine being

Since the Spirit is all in all things, the spiritual person honors and cherishes life, thus living more and more in the inner truth which makes him free. And so, the one who wants to find the inner truth that makes him free has to recognize and go through the law of cause and effect, of sowing and reaping — and, when necessary, suffer through it.

Man is called upon to gradually give up his humanness, that is, his opinions, conceptions and theories, all his ego-centricity, in order to be able to merge into the divine.

The soul incarnates so that in the brevity of years it may overcome what is often not possible for the soul to overcome in unimaginably long spans of light.

Through the Redeemer-deed of the Son of God, the Christ-Spirit, the redeeming light of the soul, helps every person who honestly confesses his faults, gives them over to the Inner Light and strives henceforth to sin no more, neither in his sensations, feelings, thinking and acting, nor in his way of speaking.

The laws of evolution are found in the law of cause and effect, the causal law

The law of cause and effect, the causal law, merges into the eternal law, into the primordial law, God.

The one who has found his way out of the causal law by purging and purifying his soul approaches the union with the All-Highest. And so, every burdened soul has to go through the causal law in order to again become as perfect as the Father in heaven.

Only the souls and people who have reached the higher steps towards perfection will love each other selflessly more and more.

On higher levels of consciousness the bond of selfless love will also be the strength in marriage and partnership that unites two people in freedom and selflessness with God, their eternal Father, thus enabling them to walk together to the Absoluteness, to the Godhead.

People who are on the higher steps towards perfection see their being together as a community with God.

Because of their lawful way of thinking and living, they feel integrated into the great family of God and they live with all those who are in the light of truth.

And so, if the motives of a relationship are noble and pure, God-pleasing, then there will no longer be quarreling and fighting, but rather a mutual understanding and confidence.

Trust in marriage and partnership is the basis for selfless love

Only an absolute mutual confidence between both partners that is based on selflessness makes it possible to have an inner openness towards all human beings who think and live in a similar way.

Confidence expresses trust. I trust her or him. If I trust a person then I set him free from within; I leave him his free will.

A person cannot breathe and flourish under coercion and pressure, but only in freedom and peace. Depending on his degree of selfless love, a person is free from bindings and opinions.

The way a person is internally is also how he influences his neighbor. If he is still tied to people and things, then he will also tie his partner to himself. If he is free of the opinions and conceptions of his neighbor, if he does not allow them to be forced upon him, but thinks about them clearly and with concentration, he will let his neighbor be free and give him his trust.

The person who loves selflessly gives his neighbor his own freedom, since he himself is free. The one who loves selflessly also has confidence in his neighbor, no matter whether the latter appreciates or disregards it.

Selfless love is spiritual greatness.

The one who knows and lives in the truth knows that the principle of equality is contained in the law of the heavens, which says: like draws to like again and again.

Similarly vibrating higher forces complement and support each other; they do not hold and bind each other. A person who wants to keep his neighbor will lose him.

The one who has climbed the ladder of evolution and, to a large extent, is in the Absolute Law, God, sees all people, the worldly ones and the spiritual ones, as they really are.

He sees them with the eyes of the spirit and knows how to place his neighbor, how he should approach him, what to say or what not to say, on the basis of his spiritual consciousness.

Every person shows who he is, the spiritual man and the worldly man

The condition of a person's inner state, his way of thinking, living and acting, his behavior and conduct, his way of talking, his manners and customs, his clothes and his home, all show who he is.

People who strive solely for worldly things, who look for a hold in passions and cravings in an undisciplined manner are unfree people who, in turn, influence their neighbor according to their own desires and wants, making them their slaves insofar as these are servile to them.

Unfree people become resigned very quickly if they do not get what is their every thought and want. Each resignation leads to discontentment and greediness.

The one who is resigned and dissatisfied with what he has, making other people responsible for it, will not receive more. Rather, he will lose even more.

Inner and outer contentedness is a sign of true spirituality. Such people will not lack anything; they will not live in excess, but will possess what they need and even more if this is good for them.

When a person lacks tolerance and generosity — generally speaking, the divine aspects — then he is or will become weak.

People who aim for worldly things alone need a great deal of physical strength. They do not receive the physical energies from the spiritual potential of the soul, but need to provide themselves with these in increased measure through food, stimulants and drugs.

And so, the one who possesses little spirituality will consume food, stimulants, medicines and the like in extra large quantities. What is not released by the inner self, by the spiritual energy, has to be replaced externally, that is, by too much food, stimulants and the like. But the external intake of energy does not bring about health or stability for the body in the long run.

The spiritual potential of the soul bears in itself the energies that stabilize and increase one's endurance from within. Joy, harmony and selflessness flow to a person from the spheres of divine life. These energies flow increasingly into him only when he actualizes the laws of unity, peace and love little by little.

As revealed before, the energy that man receives from food and stimulants reaches its limits very quickly, depending on the degree of spirituality that a person possesses. The more spiritless a person is, that is, the farther he has moved away from the source of the wellspring, the spirit of life, the power of all Being, the weaker is his spiritual and physical energy potential.

With food, stimulants and medications, the physical body can be restored again and again over a long period of time. External occasions, too, like social events that uplift a person's mood, are ways by which he tries to fool himself about his unfulfilled life.

Many people are body-centered. They place great value on proper nutrition and on the harmonizing of their body. Such a way of thinking and acting does not bring about any resonance in the soul. The soul, the energy source for a true and healthy life, does not increase in light and strength in this way.

There is another category of people who not only take their life force from food, stimulants and the intake of medicines, but who draw the life force from their fellow man, much like vampires. The victims are those who think and live on the same or similar level of vibration and who have a weaker will than those who likewise seek their refuge in material things or people.

Such weak willed people, who make the opinions and conceptions of their neighbors their own, very often unwittingly give up a part of their own life force to those like them, who have a stronger will and with it influence the weak willed and servile.

The one who willingly lets himself be subjugated by his neighbor, who consciously affirms the opinions and conceptions of others and makes them his own, serves as a slave and at the same time as a fuel pump, so to speak, for those who force their will on him.

Like draws to like, either to stimulate and fortify each other or to subjugate the weaker willed one and to pull valuable life force from him, perhaps unknowingly. In these or similar ways, many a self-centered person restores his physical potential at the expense of those who are servile to him and who make his opinions and conceptions their own.

When people have worked on or used objects, their positive or negative energies cling to these objects. These energies can also be taken in by certain types of people who are deeply rooted in matter with their thinking and wanting.

It is especially the negative energies on people and things that offer themselves again and again to those who vibrate in the same or like way. Such low energies practically impose themselves and want to establish communication with the same kinds of energies by whatever means. People who are very materialistically inclined are the magnets for these energies.

Another possibility to charge up the external magnetic field alone, is when people are uplifted by their possessions, boosting their will for further earthly aims, or when they attract the energies which their neighbor has transferred to their possessions by touching them, by living in the rooms and touching the furniture.

Every object gradually becomes charged with the energies of the person who frequently uses it. And so, there are several possibilities by which a person biased towards the world can repeatedly charge his energy potential. He can draw energy from objects, things and people, in order to charge his own weak energy field.

When the same or like vibrations meet, they communicate with each other; they stimulate and fortify each other, if it is in a higher frequency level of vibration. The negative, lower vibrations are like vampires that try again and again to pull and drag on more highly vibrating energy fields.

A person with a weak energy field automatically draws energies from wherever they are offered to him by various circumstances.

For example, energies can be drawn from a person with a more highly vibrating energy potential in a moment of tiredness, when he does not withdraw, despite his fatigue, in order to tank up from the indwelling energy potential in him.

When a vigorous person exceeds the span of increased life force flowing to him, it is possible that his vibration will fall so low that people or souls with weaker energies and who are aligned with matter can draw from his energies in spite of his energy deficit.

When a person with a high spiritual potential runs into external difficulties that he does not recognize and clear up in time, then negative powers will pull him down more and more and he will become the victim of these low-vibrating energy fields which emanate from people and souls who consider their fellow man as fuel pumps of energy. But thought forms, too, which then influence such a person, can also draw energies from him.

Thought forms are the product of the same or like thoughts which are thought over and over. They are fog-like formations which also surround those who think and speak in the same or similar way. When, for instance, a person gets upset with his fellow man, it is possible that his energy potential declines very rapidly and that equally or similarly vibrating energy fields influence him.

People who are subject to strong emotional fluctuations, who are torn this way and that, who strive towards higher ideals and values one day and then are caught up again in matter the next, are similar to fuel pumps from which life forces are drawn.

Spiritually awakened people who are above the fate and the things of this world will neither give away energy nor let it be taken from them, even when they are helping and serving their neighbor. People of the spirit draw from the inexhaustible source, from God, who gives abundantly to those who have turned to higher ideals and values, who recognize the spiritual life as the true eternal existence and as their true being.

People of the spirit may well be tired from physical work but they are never spiritually exhausted or weakened. In few hours, during which soul and body rest, their physical strength is built up again, since they draw from the eternal source, God, which flows in the innermost part of the soul and upon which they have built their every thought and aspiration.

The Spirit, God, flows through soul and person to the same extent that the person thinks and lives in the divine. Praying for strength alone is not enough. The person has to gradually fulfill the laws of God, so that the inner source, the Spirit, can begin to flow more intensively. In order to let this happen, the constant alignment of soul and person with the highest source, with God, is necessary in his thinking, wanting and acting.

The eternal power does not give of itself for selfish purposes. It may very well maintain soul and person, but does not give more than this for the human longings, desires, cravings and passions, for increasing earthly wealth and for prestige.

People who live with and in the world, whose every striving and aspiration is oriented towards the world, need, as revealed before, plenty of food, including luxuries and stimulants. They need these because the energies of God do not flow to them in the measure to which they give away their life and physical energies.

This is why people who are only materialistic will become pleasure-seeking people who devour their food — which they cannot get enough of. For this reason, food is offered in many variations and forms in order to satisfy the spoiled palate of man as well as his pleasure-seeking drives and to appease his ravenous appetite.

Because of unlawful, negative thinking, speaking and acting, a great deal of life force and physical energy is wasted by people who are oriented towards the world. An active sexual life also plays an important role in this problem. Through it, energies are discharged which in time unimaginably weaken the body and make man a slave to his desires and passions. In order to replace the energies used up in excess, he tries to regain them through widely varied and rich foods, as well as through stimulants and drugs.

The more physical energy a person wastes with unnecessary thoughts, words and actions as well as through his sexual activities, the more impoverished he becomes in spiritual strength. If he does not fulfill the law of life, his inner light, his spiritual strength, becomes ever weaker. The effects of this then cause, in turn, a greater intake of food, stimulants, medicines and the like.

In this way, man falls into ever lower levels of the human ego, until he has reached the threshold of the animal-man and in some cases he is even below this. If soul and man have little spiritual energy, the person tries to compensate for this in other ways. By so doing, he forgets who he is, namely a being of divine origin.

In this way, man becomes a robber of nature in order to satisfy his cravings and refill the lacking energy potential of his body. Because of these low human stirrings and inclinations, the body then craves animal products more and more.

The lower the spiritual potential of the soul, the more the person craves animal foods, especially meat and fish products.

To the same extent that a person has more or less — depending on his consciousness — deadened his feelings towards all life forms and thinks only of his own well-being, in the same way his behavior becomes coarse and savage. He kills animals because his world of feelings for these life forms has become disturbed.

Man does not recognize himself any longer as a child of God who bears all life forms within as spiritual essence. And so the person whose best friend is himself alone, very often is brutal towards the forms of being in the mineral and plant kingdoms. He thinks only of himself, sees only his interests and leads an excessive, unrestrained life in order to support his well-being, to indulge in his lusts and to satisfy his cravings, regardless of whether his neighbor, his fellow man and also his second neighbors, the animals and plants, suffer.

The one who is not bothered by all this can be sure that his consciousness is disturbed. He has little understanding for his fellow man and just as little for the creatures in the forests and fields, neither does he understand other forms of life, the plants and minerals.

Whatever the worldly person needs for himself he takes to the extent it is possible, without thought or question regarding the way he demands it from the earth and nature and how they cope with this.

What the world-oriented man needs for his own purposes, as support and echo, are people of his own character

He feels comfortable only when he is among those of like mind and when he receives confirmation from them. Together with them, he wants to dominate those whose nature is different from his.

Since a great many people are like him, believing in themselves and in God, but only in an intellectual way, they can hardly understand people of the spirit. To them they are eccentrics, or even described as unworldly, because they do not behave and show themselves as the masses do. Especially the person who is caught up by the world in particular will give little thought to whether h i s pattern of thinking may be wrong. He bases himself on the large number of people who think like he does.

89

The one who observes the masses, who sees them through spiritual eyes, recognizes that many people are suffering, that they are frightened and demanding, that they are marked by need, illness and worry, and that their life is disharmonious and full of quarrels and disputes.

However, the one who observes the spiritual man on the path of evolution can see the gradual ennoblement of the inner and outer being. He recognizes the changes that result from striving towards higher ethics and morals. He can feel the power that flows to people of the spirit, because they live by higher ideals and values. He will realize that the alignment with the Highest brings a raising of the consciousness.

In terms of their consciousness, people of the spirit are above the people of the world. The worldly man feels this very well. This is why he often looks down upon the one who strives for higher ideals with pity, as he cannot understand him because of his lower spiritual development.

People of the spirit see their neighbor as he truly is.

The one who refines his senses and ennobles his way of thinking, speaking and acting attains a finer body-structure, a fine vibration.

Every human body is, like everything else, radiation. Every life form is radiation. Melodious sound flows from it, all in accordance with the degree of consciousness to which the life form belongs.

The finer the radiation of a person is, the purer is his soul

Soul and person also have their sound. The sound of the human body is according to the state of consciousness of the person. This sound is audible: the person's words, the way he speaks, which words he uses, all indicate his mental-spiritual development. The way a person speaks and his choice of words indicate the melody of his body.

The shape of a person's body, his clothing and his expression also indicate what kind of spirit rules him, giving witness to who he is. And so, his way of thinking, speaking, acting and expressing himself indicates the sound of his body.

Many people try to conceal their coarse vibration, the dissonances of their body-sound, by hiding their true nature behind the mask of affectation and artificiality. By so doing, they want to be more than they actually are. The one veils over his character and thinks he can hide the dissonances behind his mask of pretended friendliness.

The other gives free rein to his character. The truly wise person recognizes both of them. The depths of the human ego are hidden only to those who still think and live in a human way.

However, everything is evident to the truly wise one, who is rich in his inner being. To him, the worldly person who shows himself other than he is, is an open book. The wise eye sees through the person of the world and recognizes the condition of the latter's consciousness immediately. Consequently, the truly enlightened person knows who he is dealing with and how he should act towards him.

Whether a person is rich or poor, whether he has cultivated table manners or not, no matter how he conducts himself, he always shows who he is.

Every exaggeration, every artificiality indicates the state of a person's consciousness — in his conduct as well as in his choice of food, his table manners or in his social life. Everything that has not grown from within, from the origin of the soul, that is, everything that is not spiritual wealth in a person, is unnatural and acquired.

Wherever it is not the spiritual in man that dominates, but the ego, the human will, there is neither freedom nor the radiating power of selflessness.

Man is deformed in his nature, confined by his ego, because he wants something only for himself, often without regard for his neighbor.

Recognize yourself at the table: How you dine and what you eat shows who you are.

The one whose main nutrition consists of spicy foods, meat and fish has not overcome his animal nature and his compulsive drives. According to his state of consciousness, his spiritual and physical attitude, a person reaches for what he himself still is. His thoughts and words, his cravings and passions, also mark his choice of food and beverages.

Spicy foods and strong alcoholic drinks show that the person who still prefers these things will also be implacable in his way of thinking, speaking and acting towards his fellow man. The sharpness of his nature, the harshness of his character, is expressed in his choice of food as well as in his table manners and in his social behavior.

His clothes and his home also bear witness of his character. A negligent character will, for example, gulp down the food at the table, talk with a full mouth and drink beverages while his mouth is still full of food. At the same time he speaks and gesticulates to emphasize his words.

The way a person takes in his food, the way he eats and dines, also shows how he acts towards his fellow man, if not externally then certainly in his thoughts.

He will encounter his neighbor like he takes in his food or gulps it down.

A person of coarse build, whose table manners are either not aesthetic or aesthetic only insofar as they are acquired, will treat his neighbor in the world similarly as he treats food at the table.

Just as he dissects the meat with knife and fork, tearing it briefly with his teeth and then swallowing it down and thus feeding his body, in a like manner will he treat his fellow man.

He will more or less tear them apart in his thoughts and with words, and if he could, he would most of all like to tear them into little pieces.

Thus, what you are can be seen in your conduct, in your way of thinking and acting.

Your facial expression as well and the shape of your body, your posture, every gesture, your countenance, the way you walk, the overall impression of your person, all show what kind of spirit rules you.

Your disharmonious gestures and your heavy gait point to the disharmony of your soul, to inner difficulties and external problems. A heavy gait also indicates a burdened soul that has to expiate many a thing that still lies latent in it.

Men of little spiritual mobility are also physically immobile and inflexible in their thinking

A person's inflexibility indicates, in turn, a strong egocentricity, an attachment to one's own pattern of thinking, which is his own conceptions and opinions.

The inflexibility of the human ego has many variations. Just to mention a few:

The inflexible person is usually rigidly tied to his conceptions, especially when his intellect is his hobby. Fanaticism is also a side branch of inflexibility. The person wants to attain something that has not yet grown in or from him.

Externally he acquires something which he thinks is good and right, but internally it often looks different. The person is inconsistent and undecided. He then tries to cover up what he actually is with harshness.

Such people often dress in a very conspicuous way and deck themselves out with a lot of jewelry. In this way, they want to inflate themselves.

Every self-inflating act of a person indicates little self-confidence. Thus, he has not yet overcome himself. In many cases such people are imitators, who live as vegetarians where their health is concerned, but are not true vegetarians.

I call them body-oriented vegetarians or body-vegetarians. Contrary to the spiritually awakened man, the spiritual vegetarian, they are interested solely in their body, in their physical health. They do not act out of responsibility for, and unity with, their second neighbor.

People of the spirit are conquerors of their base thoughts

This results in a love for creation, for all life forms. Thus, their character is ennobled. Their radiation becomes fine.

Because of finer, nobler thoughts, the fine radiation of the body, they reject meat and fish as food, because their second neighbors would have to be killed for this.

The one who first overcomes his base nature, his negative thoughts, feelings, stirrings, inclinations and physical drives attains a fine radiation. Because of his spiritual transformation he will also choose his food accordingly.

The principles of spiritual ethics and morals are the ideals and values of people on higher levels of consciousness. They treat all forms of life as they want their neighbor to treat them

After all, who wants his neighbor to beat and speak evil of him? Who wants to be driven from his homeland or his present destination in this world by force?

Who wants to be abused, maltreated or even killed by his neighbor? What you, the human being, do not want to be done to you is what you should not do to your neighbor and second neighbor and to the nature kingdoms.

Nature gives itself to man in its multiplicity and abundance.

The one who thinks of his own interests less and less and starts thinking more of life in the great totality is the one who strives for high ethics and morals. And he accepts the gifts of nature thankfully. This is the person of fine radiation. Such people will not maltreat the earth, but will prepare it at the proper time so that healthy growth may come forth from it.

Every one has to one day experience the transformation from a base nature to a divine being. No coarse build, no low vibration, no burdened soul will enter the glory of God.

Only the noble being, the pure radiating spirit body which has gained high ethics and morals in the human garment— through an ethical, virtuous life, through noble, selfless thoughts, through pure words and selfless deeds — can enter the glory of God.

These attributes of a spiritual person can also be seen in his gestures, in his facial expressions, in the shape of his body, in his clothing, in his home. And: How he dines and what he eats shows who he is.

* * *

May this short exposition, this small reference book, give each reader insight into what and who he is.

The best wishes from the divine world go with him.

The guidance of God is direct for every one who has truly ennobled his being and spiritualized his nature.

A true, noble humanity awakens on the basis of spiritual thinking and acting, not on the basis of fanaticism. Through this, the consciousness expands. Soul and man ennoble themselves and gradually become one with the divine.

Greetings in God

Brother Emanuel,
the cherub of divine Wisdom

Appendix

What Is Universal Life

Universal Life can be compared with a great and mighty tree.

Its life grew out of a little seed that was planted in the acre of this world: the revelations of the Eternal, of the Christ-of-God, that first took place before a small circle of Christ-friends.

The seed sprouted and became a small seedling that already showed what was hidden within its core: God's light, that is, love and wisdom.

As this little seedling grew, it brought further light: the Homebringing Mission of Jesus Christ with the first instructions of the Christ-of-God for a divine life among men.

This work of teaching and explanation that was called into life by the Christ-of-God eighteen years ago quickly grew into a strong plant, a small tree that was rooted in God's love and wisdom: All the basic wisdom of life was given to us men, so that we can find the way into a God-life that brings forth its fruits.

Ever more people drank from the well of divine revelations, and the little tree became a tree of life. People gathered to fulfill the will of God. And so, from the small seed that bore the life, God, grew the great and mighty tree of life called Universal Life, meaning: living in the Spirit of God, living not only for the individual but for all who are of good will.

The root of this work of God — Christ in His divine revelations given over a period of over 20 years — has reached millions of people, thus fulfilling what Jesus commanded of His own: to bear the gospel of love into all the world. Two thousand years ago Jesus said the following: "When the Spirit of truth comes, he will guide you into all truth." In our time of change, He is come and guides us into all truth — insofar as we can understand His words and receive them into our consciousness.

Now, the fruit of the deed is ripening on the great and mighty crown of the tree of Universal Life. It is the work of God through all those who, attracted by the great light-force of Christ, found their way to those who are building this work of life together. It is a small people, a people in Christ that is emerging for Christ, for a new world under the sign of love and wisdom and of peace, upright men and women who daily live more and more in His Spirit. It is all those who say yes at every moment to the great Spirit of unity, of peace and of love, thus making it possible for the work of the Lord to spread worldwide in few years. It is all those who feel called to put into practice God's love and wisdom in community. Daily, they are active for the higher values of life, for the Kingdom of Peace, the Kingdom of God on this earth, that was announced already by Jehovah, and for which all Christians pray in the Lord's Prayer.

The Inner Path
"Nearer, My God, to Thee"

"Follow Me" said Jesus of Nazareth. This is a clear challenge which at the same time brings up the question: How can we do this today in the 20th century? The Spirit of the Christ of God teaches the Inner Path in Universal Life, so that we people can find our way to a positive, meaningful life in God. We come to know ourselves, the positive characteristics, but also the human weaknesses. We develop independence, straightforwardness and understanding for our neighbor and overcome frustrations, aggressions, fears and their causes step by step — we practically become our own psychologist. Above all, we experience that we are never alone, but that God is near us and stands by us at all times. With Him, we are able to better master the situations of our life more and more. Through the consistent work on ourselves by mastering our faults and weaknesses with the power of the Christ of God, the Inner Path leads to a life of love for God and neighbor, to the unity with God.

For a free catalog of all our books,
cassettes and videos,
please contact:

Gabriele Publishing House
P.O. Box 2221, Deering, NH 03244
(844) 576-0937
WhatsApp/Messenger: +49 151 1883 8742
www.Gabriele-Publishing-House.com

Verlag DAS WORT GmbH
im Universellen Leben
Max-Braun-Strasse 2
97828 Marktheidenfeld/Altfeld, Germany
Tel. 9391-504-132 • Fax 9391-504-133

E-mail: info@universelles-leben.org